94 Meal and Juice Recipes for Pregnant Mothers:

The Expecting Mother's Guide to Smart Nutrition

By

Joe Correa CSN

COPYRIGHT

ACKNOWLEDGEMENTS

This book is dedicated to my friends and family that have had mild or serious illnesses so that you may find a solution and make the necessary changes in your life.

94 Meal and Juice Recipes for Pregnant Mothers:

The Expecting Mother's Guide to Smart Nutrition

By

Joe Correa CSN

CONTENTS

ABOUT THE AUTHOR

After years of Research, I honestly believe in the positive effects that proper nutrition can have over the body and mind. My knowledge and experience has helped me live healthier throughout the years and which I have shared with family and friends. The more you know about eating and drinking healthier, the sooner you will want to change your life and eating habits.

Nutrition is a key part in the process of being healthy and living longer so get started today. The first step is the most important and the most significant.

INTRODUCTION

94 Meal and Juice Recipes for Pregnant Mothers: The Expecting Mother's Guide to Smart Nutrition

By Joe Correa CSN

Some studies show that pregnant women need more protein, calcium, iron, and folic acid. These nutrients should come from a healthy and well-balanced diet. Your proteins should come from healthy sources like lean meat, fish, poultry, eggs, legumes, and nuts. You have to keep in mind that proteins are "builder nutrients" and are crucial for organ development, especially the brain and heart.

Your body is in a state of constant change and that is completely normal. These changes vary from mood swings caused by hormonal imbalances to morning sickness, and the obvious physical changes that occur in your body. A proper diet is definitely the best thing you can do for yourself at this moment. Don't become the victim of your cravings. Most women fall into the trap of sugar cravings. This will cause even more hormonal imbalances. Instead of candy, choose a healthier option, such as a fruit, since this help you get the right vitamins you and your baby need.

These pregnancy meal and juice recipes were created to

help you improve your nutrition during and after pregnancy. Enjoy every recipe during this joyous and exciting time in your life.

94 MEAL AND JUICE RECIPES FOR PREGNANT MOTHERS: THE EXPECTING MOTHER'S GUIDE TO SMART NUTRITION

MEALS

1.   Pumpkin Chocolate Bars

Ingredients:

2 large eggs, beaten

½ cup of oil

18 oz of yellow cake mix, (1 package)

1 tsp of pumpkin pie spice

1 cup of dark chocolate, melted

½ cup of almonds, chopped

1 tbsp of pumpkin seeds

Preparation:

Preheat the oven to 350°F.

Combine the oil and eggs in mixing bowl. Stir in the cake mix and pumpkin pie spice until well mixed.

Fold in chocolate, almonds, and pumpkin seeds. Shape the bars and spread into greased a baking dish and bake for 20-30 minutes. remove from the oven and cut into desired sizes. Serve with yogurt or homemade fruit jam.

Nutrition information per serving: Kcal: 227, Protein: 3.0g, Carbs: 25.6g, Fats: 12.8g

2. Kiwi Blueberry Smoothie

Ingredients:

½ cup of blueberries

1 medium-sized kiwi, peeled and chopped

½ medium-sized banana, sliced

1 small apricot, chopped

½ cup of Greek yogurt

1 tbsp of honey, pasteurized

¼ tsp of cinnamon, ground

Preparation:

Combine all ingredients in a blender. Blend until nicely smooth and transfer to a serving glasses. Refrigerate for 1 hour before serving.

Nutrition information per serving: Kcal: 149, Protein: 6.3g, Carbs: 30.4g, Fats: 1.6g

3.   Whole Grain Muffins

Ingredients:

1 cup of almond milk

½ cup of applesauce, unsweetened

¼ cup of maple syrup

1 cup of cornmeal

1 cup of corn

1 cup of oat flour

1 tsp of baking powder

1 tsp of baking soda

1 tbsp of flaxseeds

¼ tsp of salt

Preparation:

Preheat the oven to 375°F.

Combine almond milk and flaxseeds in a small bowl. Set aside and let it soak for about 5-7 minutes.

Combine oat flour, baking powder, baking soda, cornmeal, and salt in a large bowl. Stir in applesauce and maple syrup.

Pour the almond milk mixture and add corn. Give it a good stir until well combined.

Spoon the mixture into muffin molds or cups. Place it in the oven and bake for about 20 minutes. Insert a toothpick in the center and if it comes clean, it's done. Repeat this several times after 15 minutes of baking. Remove from the oven and serve.

Nutrition information per serving: Kcal: 179, Protein: 3.4g, Carbs: 27.0g, Fats: 7.2g

4. Cheesy Spinach & Tomato Omelet

Ingredients:

4 large eggs, beaten

½ cup of cottage cheese

½ cup of onion, finely chopped

1 cup of fresh spinach, finely chopped

6 cherry tomatoes, diced

1 tbsp of butter

½ tsp of salt

¼ tsp of black pepper, ground

Preparation:

Melt the butter in a nonstick skillet over a medium-high temperature. Add onions and cook until soften. Add eggs and spread evenly with a spatula. Cook for 3 minutes, or until bottom lightly browned.

Spread the cheese, spinach and tomatoes on one half of the pan. Sprinkle with salt and pepper to taste and fold the omelet to cover the veggies. Reduce the heat to low and cook for 2 more minutes. Remove from the heat and transfer the omelet to a serving plate. Top with extra cheese and serve!

Nutrition information per serving: Kcal: 131, Protein: 9.8g, Carbs: 8.2g, Fats: 7.0g

5.   Curry Lentils

Ingredients:

1 cup of lentils, soaked and pre-cooked

1 cup of low fat cream

4 cups of water

¼ tsp of salt

½ tsp of coriander, ground

½ tsp of Cayenne pepper, ground

¼ tsp of turmeric, ground

1 tsp of cumin, ground

1 small onion, chopped

2 tbsp of butter

1 tbsp of Chinese parsley, chopped

Preparation:

Soak lentils in cool water for at least 1 hour. The best option is to soak overnight.

Pour water in a large saucepan and bring to a boil, then turn the heat to medium-low. Rinse lentils well and add to the pot. Stir in garlic, salt, coriander, pepper, and turmeric. Cover with a lid and cook for 40 minutes, or until lentils are tender. Add more water if needed.

Melt the butter in nonstick skillet over a medium-low temperature. Add chopped onion and cook until golden brown. Stir in cumin, and fry about 1-2 minutes. Stir constantly.

Now, stir in the onions and butter into the lentils; cook on low heat for another 5-8 minutes. Add low fat cream and allow it to melt. Garnish with chopped parsley and serve.

Nutrition information per serving: Kcal: 179, Protein: 8.8g, Carbs: 21.9g, Fats: 6.5g

6.   Choco Avocado Mousse

Ingredients:

2 medium-sized avocados, pitted, peeled, and chopped

1 medium-sized banana, chopped

½ cup of cocoa powder, raw

5 tbsp of coconut milk

2 tbsp of maple syrup

1 tsp of vanilla extract

½ tsp of cinnamon, ground

¼ tsp of black pepper, ground

1 tsp of orange zest

Preparation:

Combine all ingredients in a food processor. Blend until nicely smooth and transfer to a serving bowls. Garnish with orange zest and serve. You can use the mousse up to 2 days in the refrigerator.

Nutrition information per serving: Kcal: 439, Protein: 6.2g, Carbs: 34.1g, Fats: 34.1g

7.   Hindu Chia Seeds

Ingredients:

1 cup of chia seeds

1 cup of low fat cream

2 garlic cloves, chopped

1 tsp of ginger, ground

¼ tsp of salt

2 small chili peppers, chopped

1 small onion, chopped

Preparation:

Pour 3 cups of water in a deep pot and bring it to a boil. Place chia seeds in and cook for 30 minutes over a low temperature, or until tender.

Add spices and mix well. Cook for about 5-10 minutes, stirring constantly. Top with low fat cream and serve.

Nutrition information per serving: Kcal: 512, Protein: 18.8g, Carbs: 46.5g, Fats: 34.4g

8.   Chickpea & Chili Soup

Ingredients:

2 tsp of cumin seeds

½ cup of chili flakes

½ cup of lentils

1 tbsp of olive oil

1 red onion , chopped

3 cups of vegetable stock

1 cup of tomatoes, chopped

½ cup of chickpeas

¼ cup of coriander, roughly chopped

4 tbsp of Greek yogurt

Preparation:

Preheat a large nonstick saucepan and add cumin seeds and chili flakes. Fry until they start to jump around the pan and release aromas.

Add the oil and onion, and cook for 5 minutes. Stir in the lentils, stock, and tomatoes. Bring to a boil and simmer for

15 minutes until lentils soften.

Transfer the soup to a blender or in a food processor. Blend until smooth and pour back into the pan. Add the chickpeas and heat gently. Season well and stir in the coriander. Finish with a dollop of yogurt and coriander leaves.

Serve warm.

Nutrition information per serving: Kcal: 263, Protein: 15.9g, Carbs: 37.1g, Fats: 6.4g

9.   Arugula Quinoa Salad

Ingredients:

4 cups of arugula, trimmed and chopped

2 cups of white quinoa, pre-cooked

1 large bell pepper, chopped

1 small onion, chopped

1 cup of cherry tomatoes, halved

2 tbsp of almonds, toasted and chopped

¼ cup of orange juice

¼ cup of lemon juice

¼ cup of balsamic vinegar

½ tsp of sea salt

¼ tsp of black pepper, ground

3 cups of water

Preparation:

Combine orange juice, lemon juice, vinegar, sea salt, and pepper to a mixing bowl. Stir well and set aside to allow flavors to meld.

Combine quinoa and water in a deep pot. Bring it to a boil and cook for 20 minutes, or until tender. Remove from the heat and rinse with cold water. Drain well and transfer to a large bowl. Add arugula, pepper, and tomatoes. Drizzle with dressing and toss well to coat. Sprinkle with toasted almonds.

Refrigerate for at least 1 hour before serving.

Nutrition information per serving: Kcal: 187, Protein: 7.1g, Carbs: 31.9g, Fats: 3.6g

10.   Fried Egg Whites with Cottage Cheese

Ingredients:

4 large eggs, beaten

1 cup of cottage cheese

¼ cup of skim milk

1 tbsp of olive oil

1 tsp of salt

Preparation:

Remove the egg whites from yolks and set aside.

Preheat the oil on a nonstick frying pan over a medium-high temperature.

Meanwhile, whisk together egg whites, cottage cheese and milk. Sprinkle with some salt to taste. Pour the mixture into the pan and fry for about 3-4 minutes, stirring constantly. Remove from the pan and sprinkle with some fresh parsley for extra taste. Serve immediately.

Nutrition information per serving: Kcal: 316, Protein: 29.1g, Carbs: 6.4g, Fats: 19.1g

11. Legumes on Mexican Way

Ingredients:

½ cup of white beans

½ cup of black beans

½ cup of green peas

½ cup of green beans

1 tsp of red chili powder

2 tbsp of all-purpose flour

1 tbsp of onion powder

½ tsp of dried oregano, ground

½ tsp of garlic powder

½ tsp of cumin, ground

½ tsp of salt

3 cups of water

Preparation:

Place the legumes in a deep bowl. Add water to cover all ingredients. Soak overnight.

Drain well and place in a deep pot. Add 3 cups of water and bring it to a boil. Cook for 25 minutes, then add all other ingredients. Reduce the heat to low and cover with a lid. Cook for another 20 minutes. Remove from the heat and serve.

Nutrition information per serving: Kcal: 169, Protein: 10.5g, Carbs: 31.3g, Fats: 0.7g

12.   Apple Spinach Smoothie

Ingredients:

1 cup of fresh spinach, chopped

1 small apple, cored and chopped

1 large pear, cored and chopped

½ cup of water

3 tbsp of lemon juice

1 tbsp of orange juice

2 tbsp of honey

Preparation:

Combine all ingredients in a food processor. Blend until smooth and transfer to a serving glasses. Add a few ice cubes and serve, or refrigerate 1 hour before serving.

Nutrition information per serving: Kcal: 245, Protein: 1.3g, Carbs: 45.1g, Fats: 0.6g

13.   Cold Cauliflower Salad

Ingredients:

1 lb cauliflower florets

1 lb broccoli

2 medium-sized chicken fillets, cut into bite-sized pieces

4 garlic cloves, crushed

¼ cup of extra virgin olive oil

1 tsp of salt

1 tbsp of dry rosemary, crushed

Preparation:

Rinse and drain the vegetables. Cut into bite-sized pieces.

Preheat the olive oil over a medium-high heat and add crushed garlic. Stir-fry for 1-2 minutes, then add cauliflower, broccoli, chicken fillets, and about ½ cup of water. Reduce the heat to minimum and simmer until fork-tender.

When the most of the liquid has evaporated, add salt and crushed rosemary. Give it a good stir and remove from the heat.

Allow it to cool well in the refrigerator before serving.

Nutrition information per serving: Kcal: 182, Protein: 25.7g, Carbs: 15.1g, Fats: 13.2g

14.   Cumin Chicken

Ingredients:

8 oz chicken thighs, cut into bite-sized pieces

4 tbsp of honey, pasteurized

1 tbsp of dry oregano

2 tbsp of coconut oil

1 tsp of cumin, ground

1 tsp of sea salt

1 tsp of black pepper, ground

1 tbsp of fresh mint, chopped

Preparation:

Preheat the oil in a large skillet over a medium-high temperature.

Add chicken and cook for 8 minutes or until golden brown. Add onion and toss for another 3 minutes. Sprinkle with salt, pepper, oregano and cumin to taste. Stir in honey and cinnamon.

Toss for about 5 minutes more and cook until heated through.

Garnish with mint and serve hot.

Nutrition information per serving: Kcal: 170, Protein: 38.5g, Carbs: 11.2g, Fats: 21.4g

15.   Oatmeal Mango Cream

Ingredients:

2 cups of mango, peeled and chopped

3 tbsp of oatmeal

2 tbsp of skim milk

2 tbsp of Greek yogurt

1 tbsp of flaxseeds

Preparation:

Using package instructions, prepare oatmeal. Set aside.

Place mango in a food processor and blend until smooth. Transfer to a medium bowl and stir in milk, yogurt, and flaxseeds. Garnish with mint or berries.

Nutrition information per serving: Kcal: 269, Protein: 7.0g, Carbs: 57.8g, Fats: 3.3g

16.   Beef Moussaka

Ingredients:

2 lb large potatoes, peeled and sliced

1 lb lean ground beef

1 large onion, peeled and finely chopped

1 tsp of salt

½ tsp of black pepper, ground

½ cup of milk

2 large eggs, beaten

Vegetable oil

Sour cream or Greek yogurt, for serving

Preparation:

Preheat the oven to 400 degrees.

Grease the bottom of a 8x8 inches baking dish with some vegetable oil. Make one layer with sliced potatoes and brush with some milk. Spread the ground beef and make another layer with potatoes. Brush well with the remaining milk, add ½ cup of water, and close the lid.

Cook for one hour, or until the potatoes are completely soft.

When done, make the final layer with beaten egg. Bake for another ten minutes.

Top with some sour cream or Greek yogurt and serve!

Nutrition information per serving: Kcal: 458, Protein: 34.9g, Carbs: 36g, Fats: 19.2g

17.   Swiss Chard with Toasted Pine Nuts

Ingredients:

2 oz of Swiss chard, chopped

1 medium-sized yellow bell pepper, sliced

1 small green apple, cored and chopped

¼ cup of pine nuts, lightly toasted

¼ of fennel bulb, chopped into bite-sized pieces

2 tbsp of walnut oil

2 tbsp of sherry vinegar

½ tsp of salt

½ tsp of black pepper, ground

Preparation:

Mix together vinegar, salt, and pepper in a mixing bowl. Set aside.

Combine the vegetables in a large bowl. Add apple slices and pine nuts. Toss well to combine and serve.

Nutritional information per serving: Calories: 85, Protein: 2.0g Carbs: 8.8g Fats: 5.6g

18. Raw Cocoa Muffins

Ingredients:

½ cup of flaxseed, ground

2 ½ cup of almond flour

3 tsp of baking powder

6 tbsp of cocoa powder, raw

1 tsp of cinnamon, ground

2 cups of coconut milk

1 cup of honey, pasteurized

2 tsp of vanilla powder

½ cup of olive oil

1 tbsp of coconut flour

Preparation:

Preheat the oven to 375°F.

Combine all dry ingredients in a bowl. Gently whisk in the coconut milk, add the honey and oil. Mix well with an electric mixer. Shape the muffins using molds and place in paper liners.

Bake the muffins for about 15 minutes. if the inserted toothpick in the muffin comes out clean, they are done.

Sprinkle with coconut flour and cool for a while before serving.

Nutrition information per serving: Kcal: 278, Protein: 4.5g, Carbs: 48.6, Fats: 12.2g

19.   Ginger Omelet

Ingredients:

4 free-range eggs

2 tbsp of extra-virgin olive oil

1 tsp of fresh ginger, grated

¼ tsp of black pepper, ground

¼ cup of raisins

¼ tsp of sea salt

Preparation:

Beat the eggs with a fork. Sprinkle with some ginger and pepper. Whisk well to combine.

Preheat the oil in a large frying pan over a medium-high temperature. pour the egg mixture and sprinkle with some salt to taste. Cook for 4 minutes, or until set. Remove from the heat and top with raisins. Serve immediately.

Nutrition information per serving: Kcal: 608, Protein: 23.5g, Carbs: 31.7, Fats: 45.8g

20.   Leafy Greens with Walnuts

Ingredients:

2 cups of Romaine lettuce, chopped

1 large orange, peeled and wedged

¼ cup of walnuts

¼ cup of dates, pitted and finely chopped

1 tbsp of fresh lemon juice

Preparation:

Combine the ingredients in a large bowl and drizzle with lemon juice. Mix well and refrigerate for 30 minutes before serving.

Nutrition information per serving: Kcal: 148, Protein: 12.3g, Carbs: 21.6g, Fats: 8.3g

21.   Carrot Beet Booster

Ingredients:

2 large carrots, chopped

2 small beets, trimmed and chopped

1 tbsp of lemon juice

1 large orange, peeled and wedged

2 tbsp of chia seeds

Preparation:

Combine all ingredients in a food processor and blend until nicely smooth. Transfer to a serving glasses and add a few ice cubes. Garnish with more chia seeds for some extra nutrients.

Nutrition information per serving: Kcal: 122, Protein: 6.2g, Carbs: 38.1g, Fats: 9.2g

22. Stuffed Onions

Ingredients:

10-12 medium-sized sweet onions, peeled

1 lb of lean ground beef

½ cup of rice

3 tbsp of olive oil

1 tbsp of dry mint, ground

1 tsp of Cayenne pepper, ground

½ tsp of cumin, ground

1 tsp of salt

½ cup of tomato paste

½ cup bread crumbs

A handful of fresh parsley, finely chopped

Preparation:

Cut a ¼-inch slice from top of each onion and trim a small amount from the bottom end, This will make the onions stand upright. Place onions in a microwave-safe dish and add about one cup of water. Cover with a tight lid and microwave on HIGH 10 to 12 minutes or until onions are tender. Remove onions from a dish and cool slightly. Now carefully remove inner layers of onions with paring knife, leaving about a ¼-inch onion shell.

In a large bowl, combine ground beef with rice, olive oil, mint, cayenne pepper, cumin, salt, and bread crumbs. Use one tablespoon of the mixture to fill the onions.

Grease the bottom of a deep pot with some oil and add onions. Add about 2 ½ cups of water and cover. Cook for 45 minutes over medium heat.

Sprinkle with chopped parsley or even arugula and serve with sour cream or Greek yogurt.

Nutrition information per serving: Kcal: 464, Protein: 34g, Carbs: 48.4g, Fats: 15.2g

23.   Chicken Wings Stew

Ingredients:

1 lb chicken breast

2 large potatoes, peeled and finely chopped

5 large green bell peppers, finely chopped and seeds removed

2 small carrots, sliced

1 large tomato, roughly chopped

A handful of fresh parsley, finely chopped

3 tbsp of extra virgin olive oil

1 tbsp of cayenne pepper

1 tsp of freshly ground chili pepper

1 tsp of salt

Preparation:

Grease a deep pot with three tablespoons of olive oil. Place the vegetables and top with chicken wings. Add one tablespoon of cayenne pepper, salt, and a handful of fresh parsley.

Add about two cups of water, close with a lid and simmer for about two hours over a medium temperature.

Nutrition information per serving: Kcal: 325, Protein: 11.5g, Carbs: 44.5g, Fats: 12.8g

24.   Almond Stuffed Eggplants

Ingredients:

4 medium-sized eggplants, halved lengthwise

4 small onions, peeled and finely chopped

4 garlic cloves, crushed

¼ cup of parsley, finely chopped

3 medium-sized tomatoes, peeled and finely chopped

½ cup of extra-virgin olive oil

1 bay leaf, dry and crushed

2 tbsp of almonds, finely chopped

1 tbsp of honey, pasteurized

½ tsp of salt

½ tsp of black pepper, ground

Preparation:

Preheat the oven to 300°F.

Line some baking paper over a baking sheet.

Slice the eggplants in half, lengthwise. Remove the flesh

and transfer to a bowl. Add some salt and let it stand for about 30 minutes.

Preheat the oil in a large skillet over a medium-high temperature. Briefly, fry the eggplants for 3 minutes on each side and remove from the frying pan. Use some kitchen paper to soak up the excess oil. Set aside.

Add onions and garlic to the same frying pan. Stir-fry for 2 minutes and then add tomatoes. Mix well and simmer until the tomatoes soften.

Now, add the eggplant meat and the rest of the ingredients. Cook for about 5 more minutes and remove from the heat.

Stuff the eggplant halves with this mixture. Transfer to a baking dish and bake for about 15 minutes, or until lightly charred.

Serve warm with some sour cream on top, but this is optional.

Nutrition information per serving: Kcal: 219, Protein: 4.0g, Carbs: 24.4g, Fats: 14.0g

25.   Beet Apple Spinach Salad

Ingredients:

1 large beet, steamed and sliced

2 cups of spinach, trimmed

2 spring onions, finely chopped

1 small green apple, cored and stripped

¼ cup of olive oil

2 tbsp of fresh lime juice

1 tbsp of honey, pasteurized

1 garlic clove, crushed

1 tsp of apple cider vinegar

¼ tsp of black pepper, ground

¼ tsp of salt

Preparation:

Place the beet in a deep pot. Pour enough water to cover and cook for about 40 minutes, or until tender. Remove the skin and slice. Transfer to a bowl. Combine olive oil, vinegar, cider, salt, pepper, and honey. Pour over beet slices and toss to coat. Let it stand for at least 30 minutes.

Wash and pat dry the apple. Slice into thin strips and combine with beet slices, spring onions, and spinach. Add crushed garlic and mix well. Serve.

Nutrition information per serving: Kcal: 343, Protein: 2.4g, Carbs: 31.9g, Fats: 25.7g

26. Ginger Chili Chicken Thighs

Ingredients:

2 lbs of chicken thighs

1 tbsp of chili pepper, ground

16 oz of coconut water

1 tbsp of ginger, ground

1 tbsp of coriander seeds

8 garlic cloves, minced

¼ cup of fresh basil, chopped

½ tsp of salt

½ tsp of black pepper, ground

Preparation:

Place chicken thighs and garlic in a slow cooker.

Sprinkle the meat with ginger, chili, salt, and pepper. Pour the coconut water and add the fresh basil. Cover with a lid and set heat to low-medium temperature.

Cook the thighs for about 8-10 hours, or until tender. Remove from the heat and give it a good stir. Serve warm.

Nutrition information per serving: Kcal: 472, Protein: 45.9g, Carbs: 6.6g, Fats: 29.3g

27.   Farmer's Breakfast

Ingredients:

4 large eggs

1 cup of baby spinach, chopped

½ cup of Goat's cheese, crumbled

1 tbsp of extra-virgin olive oil

4 bread slices, whole-grain

¼ tsp of salt

Preparation:

Beat the eggs with a fork in a bowl. Cut goat's cheese into small cubes and add them to the bowl.

Preheat the oil in a large nonstick frying pan over a medium-high temperature. Add spinach and fry for about 3-4 minutes, or until soften. Stir in the egg and cheese mixture and fry for 3 more minutes, or until eggs are set.

Put the bread in the toaster for 2 minutes. Serve with egg, cheese, and spinach mixture.

Nutrition information per serving: Kcal: 345, Protein: 19.8g, Carbs: 11.1g, Fats: 25.1g

28. Beef Stew

Ingredients:

1 lb of lean beef, cut into bite-sized pieces

½ cup red wine vinegar

1 tbsp of butter

6 oz of tomato paste

½ cup of baby carrots, sliced

2 medium-sized sweet potatoes, peeled and chopped

1 large onion, finely chopped

1 cup of button mushrooms, chopped

½ tsp of salt

1 bay leaf

2 cups beef broth

½ cup of green peas

1 tsp of dried thyme, ground

3 garlic cloves, minced

Preparation:

Melt the butter in a skillet over a medium-high temperature. Add beef chops and fry until browned, stirring constantly.

Transfer the meat to a slow cooker and reserve the pan. Add onions to the pan and cook for 5 minutes.

Pour the wine and tomato paste in the frying pan to scoop up any remaining bits of the beef and onions.

Pour the mixture over the beef in a deep pot. Put in all the remaining ingredients and stir properly, especially if the liquid is thick. Cover with a lid and cook for about 1 hour. Stir in green peas and cook for 15 minutes more. Remove from the heat and serve.

Nutrition information per serving: Kcal: 216, Protein: 21.1g, Carbs: 19.8g, Fats: 5.6g

29.   Hawaiian Pulled Pork

Ingredients:

4 lbs of pork shoulders

1 can of crushed pineapples

2 tsp of ginger, grated

1 medium-sized carrot, sliced

1 large bell pepper, chopped

1 cup of beef broth

1 tsp of salt

Preparation:

Place the meat in a large pot. Add carrot, pepper and pineapple with all its liquid. Pour the beef broth and add water to adjust thickness if needed. Sprinkle with ginger and salt to taste. Cover with a lid and cook for 1 hour on a medium-low temperature. Remove from the heat and give it a good stir. Serve warm.

Nutrition information per serving: Kcal: 239, Protein: 43.0g, Carbs: 4.0g, Fats: 39.0g

30. Coconut Mango Smoothie

Ingredients:

1 cup of mango, chopped

½ cup of Greek yogurt

1 cup of coconut milk

1 large orange, peeled and wedged

1 tbsp of coconut flour

1 tbsp of lemon juice

1 tsp of lemon zest

Preparation:

Combine mango, yogurt, coconut milk, orange, and lemon juice in a food processor. Blend until nicely smooth and transfer to a serving glasses. Top with coconut flour and sprinkle with lemon zest for extra flavor. Refrigerate for 30 minutes before serving.

Nutrition information per serving: Kcal: 313, Protein: 6.8g, Carbs: 30.2g, Fats: 20.8g

31.   Braised Lamb Shanks

Ingredients:

2 lbs lamb shanks

1 tsp of black pepper, ground

1 tsp of sea salt

2 medium-sized carrots, chopped

¼ cup of olive oil

4 garlic cloves, minced

4 cups of marinara sauce

1 large onion, chopped

Preparation:

Place all ingredients in a slow cooker. Set the heat to low temperature and cook for 8 hours. The ideal option is to cook it overnight.

The best way to check if the lamb shanks have been cooked properly is to observe if the meat is falling off the bone. It is the truest indication that the lamb shanks are ready to for serving.

Nutrition information per serving: Kcal: 312, Protein: 27.6g, Carbs: 16.9g, Fats: 14.4g

32.   Triple-Layered Brownies

Ingredients:

20 oz of brownie mix, (1 package)

3 large eggs

¼ cup of water

½ cup of oil

1 tbsp of peanut butter

16 oz of cream cheese frosting

12 oz of milk chocolate chips

2 ½ cup of crispy rice cereal

Preparation:

Preheat the oven to 300°F.

Place brownie mix in a large bowl. Gradually stir in beaten eggs, water and oil. Shape the cookies and spread over a large greased baking pan.

Bake for about 30-35 minutes, or until nicely brown. Remove from the oven and let it cool. Now, spread the frosting over each brownie.

Melt peanut butter in a medium nonstick skillet over a medium-low temperature. And the chocolate chips and stir constantly. Remove from heat when combined.

Spread evenly over the brownies. Refrigerate for 1 hour before serving.

Nutrition information per serving: Kcal: 310, Protein: 2.7g, Carbs: 43.8g, Fats: 14.9g

33. Cream Cheese Slices

Ingredients:

2 x 8 oz of crescent rolls, separated

1lb of cream cheese, softened

1 tsp of vanilla extract

½ cup of honey, pasteurized

1 tsp of cinnamon, ground

1 egg yolk

1 egg white

Preparation:

Preheat the oven to 350°F.

Lay 1 can of the crescent rolls on a greased baking pan.

Combine cream cheese, vanilla, honey and egg yolk in a blender. Transfer this mixture to the pan and spread over the crescent rolls. Gently lay remaining crescent rolls over the cream cheese mix.

In a separate bowl, whisk the eggs white until frothy and gently pour over the dough. Sprinkle with cinnamon.

Bake for about 20-25 minutes, or until brown. Remove from the oven and let it cool. Cut into slices and serve.

Nutrition information per serving: Kcal: 299, Protein: 7.5g, Carbs: 32.6g, Fats: 16.0g

34.   Peanut Butter Oats

Ingredients:

1 cup of oats, pre-cooked

1 cup of almond milk, unsweetened

2 tbsp of peanut butter, organic

1 tbsp of strawberry syrup

1 tsp of cinnamon, ground

Preparation:

Place the ingredients in a bowl and stir well until you get a nice, smooth mixture. If necessary, add some water. Pour this mixture in a tall glasses and leave in the refrigerator overnight.

Nutrition information per serving: Kcal: 554, Protein: 12.2g, Carbs: 44.9g, Fats: 39.3g

35.   Eggs & Cheese Sandwich

Ingredients:

4 large eggs

1 cup of cottage cheese

1 tsp of dried parsley, chopped

8 thin slices of bread, whole-grain

8 Romaine lettuce leaves, whole

1 medium-sized tomato, thinly sliced

½ tsp of salt

Preparation:

Boil the eggs for 10 minutes. Allow to cool and peel them. Cut into thin slices – about 5-6 slices per each egg.

Place the lettuce leaf on a slice of bread. Layer 1 tablespoon of cheese, 1-2 tomato slices, and top with eggs.Cover with another bread slice to make a sandwich. Repeat the process with remaining ingredients. If you like, you can add more vegetables. Sprinkle with salt and serve.

Nutrition information per serving: Kcal: 177, Protein: 15.8g, Carbs: 13.1g, Fats: 6.7g

36. Greek Yogurt Protein Shake

Ingredients:

3 cups of Greek yogurt

3 egg whites

1 cup of fresh apple juice

2 tbsp of orange juice, freshly squeezed

½ cup of frozen mango, chopped

½ cup of frozen pineapple, chopped

1 tbsp of honey, pasteurized

Preparation:

Combine the ingredients in a blender and mix for 30-40 seconds. Transfer to a serving glasses and refrigerate for at least 30 minutes before serving.

Nutrition information per serving: Kcal: 204, Protein: 14.5g, Carbs: 32.4g, Fats: 2.5g

37.   Green Omelet

Ingredients:

4 large eggs

1 cup of baby spinach, chopped

1 small onion, chopped

¼ tsp of red pepper, ground

¼ tsp of sea salt

1 tbsp of Parmesan cheese, grated

1 tbsp of olive oil

Preparation:

Beat the eggs with a fork, in a large bowl. Add baby spinach and Parmesan cheese. Season with salt and pepper to taste and whisk well to combine.

Preheat the oil in large nonstick frying pan over a medium-high temperature. Pour the egg mixture and cook for about 3-4 minutes, or until eggs are set.

Serve with some raw vegetables. This is, however, optional.

Nutrition information per serving: Kcal: 271, Protein: 18.1g, Carbs: 6.2g, Fats: 20.1g

38. Asparagus Artichoke Salad

Ingredients:

6 medium artichoke hearts

1 cup of asparagus, trimmed

1 cup of button mushrooms, chopped

1 cup of cherry tomatoes, halved

1 cup of Romaine lettuce, chopped

½ cup of black olives, pitted

½ cup of green olives, pitted

3 tbsp of lemon juice

2 tbsp of butter

2 tsp of Dijon Mustard

2 garlic cloves, minced

4 tbsp of olive oil

1 tsp of sea salt

½ tsp of black pepper, ground

Preparation:

Preheat the oven to 400°F.

Mix lemon juice, mustard, garlic, 2 tablespoons of oil, salt, and pepper in a mixing bowl. Stir well to combine and set aside to allow flavors to meld.

Grease a medium baking dish with 2 tablespoons of oil. Add asparagus and sprinkle with some salt to taste. Bake it for 5 minutes and remove from the heat. Set aside.

Melt the butter in a nonstick saucepan over a medium-high temperature. Add mushrooms and cook for 5 minutes. Remove from the heat and set aside.

Combine lettuce, tomatoes, green olives, artichokes, and black olives in a large salad bowl. Add asparagus and mushrooms and toss well to combine. Drizzle with dressing and give it a good stir. Refrigerate before serving

Nutrition information per serving: Kcal: 176, Protein: 5.2g, Carbs: 16.4g, Fats: 12.1g

39.   Garlic Chicken Breasts

Ingredients:

5 lbs of chicken breasts

2 cups chicken broth

½ tsp of black pepper, ground

2 garlic cloves, minced

2 large bell peppers, chopped

1 cup of tomatoes, diced

½ tsp of salt

¼ tsp of black pepper, ground

Preparation:

Place meat in a deep pot and pour the chicken broth. Cover with a lid and cook for about 4 hours over a medium-low temperature.

Meanwhile, preheat a large nonstick saucepan over a medium-high temperature. Add garlic and stir-fry until translucent. Add peppers, tomatoes, and sprinkle some salt and pepper to taste. Cook for 2 minutes and stir in the flour. Cook for 1 more minute, then pour the mixture into the pot. Stir well to combine and add more water to adjust thickness if needed. Cook for 1 hour and remove from the heat. Stir well again and serve warm.

Nutrition information per serving: Kcal: 376, Protein: 55.9g, Carbs: 2.5g, Fats: 14.3g

40.   Ginger Peach Smoothie

Ingredients:

2 large peaches, peeled and sliced

1 cup of Greek yogurt

3 tbsp of mango juice

1 tsp of ginger, freshly grated

1 tbsp of flaxseeds

Preparation:

Combine all ingredients in a food processor and blend until nicely smooth. Add a few ice cubes and re-blend for 20 seconds. Garnish with extra fruits or seeds.

Nutrition information per serving: Kcal: 280, Protein: 7.6g, Carbs: 61.8g, Fats: 3.0g

41. Cilantro-Garlic Burgers with Parmesan

Ingredients:

2 cans of lentils, drained

3 garlic cloves, minced

½ cup of breadcrumbs

¼ cup of parmesan cheese, grated

1 egg, beaten

2 cups of water

½ cup of all-purpose flour

1 tbsp of vegetable oil

½ tsp of salt

¼ tsp of black pepper, ground

Preparation:

In a medium size bowl, mash lentils with folk then mix with garlic, breadcrumbs and cheese. Form into patties; set aside.

Whisk egg and water in medium bowl. Combine flour, salt, and pepper in another bowl. Coat each patty gently with flour mixture, then dip into egg, then coat again with flour.

Preheat the oil in a large skillet over a medium-high temperature. Fry the burgers for about 2-3 minutes on each side, or until browned.

Serve with warm bread or in a pita with cilantro, yogurt, onion, tomatoes, or whatever you like. This is, however, optional.

Nutrition information per serving: Kcal: 417, Protein: 25.6g, Carbs: 64.4g, Fats: 6.3g

42. Green Salad with Strawberries & Avocado

Ingredients:

1 cup of fresh arugula, trimmed and chopped

1 cup of fresh endive, trimmed and chopped

1 cup of fresh watercress, chopped

1 cup of fresh spinach, finely chopped

1 small cucumber, sliced

1 cup of strawberries, halved

1 cup of avocado, cubed

3 tbsp of almonds, roughly chopped

3 tbsp of olive oil

2 tbsp of balsamic vinegar

1 tsp of sea salt

¼ tsp of black pepper, ground

Preparation:

Combine oil, vinegar, salt, and pepper in a mixing bowl. Stir well and set aside.

Mix together arugula, endive, watercress, spinach, and cucumber. Gently mix in the fruits. Drizzle with dressing and toss well to coat. Sprinkle with almonds and refrigerate for 1 hour to allow flavors to mingle before serving.

Nutrition information per serving: Kcal: 222, Protein: 3.1g, Carbs: 10.6g, Fats: 20.2g

43.   Veal and Chicken Kebab

Ingredients

1 lb of lean veal cuts, chopped into bite-sized pieces

1 lb of chicken breast, boneless, skinless, and chopped into bite-sized pieces

12 oz button mushrooms, sliced

3 large carrots, sliced

2 tbsp of butter, softened

1 tbsp of olive oil

1 tbsp of cayenne pepper

1 tsp of salt

½ tsp of freshly ground black pepper

A bunch of fresh celery leaves, finely chopped

3.5 oz celery root, finely chopped

Preparation:

Grease the bottom of a heavy-bottomed pot with one tablespoon of olive oil. Now add veal chops, sliced carrot, salt, pepper, cayenne pepper, and celery root. Give it a good stir and add 2 cups of water. Cook for 35-40 minutes over a medium-high heat, or until the meat is half-cooked.

Now add chicken breast, butter, and one more cup of water. Continue to simmer for 30 more minutes, or until the meat is fully cooked and tender.

Finally, add mushrooms and celery. I personally don't like to overcook the mushrooms so about 10 more minutes over a medium-heat will be more than enough.

Serve warm.

Nutrition information per serving: Kcal: 373, Protein: 37.6g, Carbs: 11.3g, Fats: 20g

44.   Banana Nut Porridge

Ingredients:

1 large banana, sliced

2 cups of coconut milk, unsweetened

1 tsp of cinnamon, ground

½ cup of cashews, chopped

½ cup of almonds, chopped

½ cup of pecans, chopped

½ tsp of salt

Preparation:

Combine all nuts in a large mixing bowl. Add water enough to cover all ingredients. Sprinkle with some salt and leave it to soak overnight.

Drain well and rinse with cold water. Transfer the nuts to a food processor and add banana, coconut milk, and cinnamon. Blend until smooth and nicely thick.

Transfer the mixture to a nonstick saucepan. Cook for about 5 minutes on medium-high temperature. Stir occasionally. Remove from the heat and let it cool for a while. Transfer to a serving bowls and top with extra nuts if desired.

Nutrition information per serving: Kcal: 499, Protein: 8.6g, Carbs: 23.5g, Fats: 45.1g

45.   Almond Meal Pancakes

Ingredients:

1 cup almond flour

2 large eggs

½ cup water

½ tsp of baking soda

¼ tsp of salt

¼ tsp of honey, pasteurized

2 oz of butter

Preparation:

Combine flour, salt, and baking soda in a large mixing bowl. Stir well and set aside.

In a separate bowl, combine eggs, honey and 1 tablespoon of butter. Whisk until well combined.

Pour the egg mixture into the bowl with the flour mixture and mix it thoroughly until smooth. If the batter mixture is too thick, add with water and mix until the desired consistency is achieved. Cover the bowl with a cloth or lid and let it stand for 15 minutes.

Add the remaining butter to a nonstick frying pan and melt over a medium-high temperature. Spoon the batter into the pan, enough to cover the bottom part of the pan.Cook for 2 minutes or until bottom is lightly browned. Repeat the procedure with the remaining butter.

Place pancakes to a serving plate and top with honey and nuts. This is, however, optional.

Nutrition information per serving: Kcal: 168, Protein: 4.3g, Carbs: 16.3g, Fats: 9.5g

46.   Coconut Blackberry Pudding with Chia & Pistachios

Ingredients:

1 cup of almond milk

½ tsp of almond extract

½ cup of fresh blackberries, crushed

3 tbsp of chia seeds

1 tbsp of coconut, shredded

¼ cup of pistachios, chopped

Preparation:

Combine crushed blackberries, chia seeds, almond extract, almond milk and shredded coconut in a large mixing bowl. Mix the ingredients well until well combined.

Cover the bowl with a plastic wrap or lid and refrigerate for at least 12 hours before serving.

Top the pudding with chopped pistachios, or any other nuts you like.

Nutrition information per serving: Kcal: 453, Protein: 9.8g, Carbs: 21.6g, Fats: 38.1g

47.   Blueberry Breakfast Tortilla

Ingredients:

½ cup of fresh blueberries

1tbsp of butter

4 eggs, beaten

1 tsp of almond butter

¼ tsp of black pepper, ground

¼ tsp of salt

1 tsp of cinnamon, ground

Preparation:

Combine almond butter, eggs, cinnamon, and pepper in a mixing bowl. Whisk well and set aside.

Melt the butter in a medium nonstick skillet over a medium-high temperature. pour the egg mixture and cook for 3 minutes, or until set. Top with blueberries and then reduce the heat to low. Cover with a lid and cook for about 6-8 minutes.

Remove the lid and place a medium plate on top of the meal and flip the egg tortilla. Return the pan to the heat and cook for another 3-4 minutes, or until set. Remove from the heat and divide into 2 equal portions. Serve.

Nutrition information per serving: Kcal: 250, Protein: 13.2g, Carbs: 8.5g, Fats: 19.2g

48.   Chickpeas Bulgur

Ingredients:

2 cups of chickpeas, pre-cooked

2 cups of bulgur, pre-cooked

1 medium-sized zucchini, peeled and chopped

1 medium –sized squash, halved and sliced

½ cup of fresh basil, chopped

4 cups of vegetable stock

1 medium-sized onion, chopped

1 tbsp of vegetable oil

2 garlic cloves, minced

½ tsp of salt

¼ cup of black pepper, ground

1 tsp of dried thyme, minced

Preparation:

Combine bulgur and vegetable stock in a deep pot. Bring it to a boil and cook, then reduce the heat to low. Cover with a lid and cook until liquid evaporates. Set aside to cool for a while.

Place the chickpeas in a pot of boiling water. Cook until tender and remove from the heat. Drain and rinse and set aside.

Preheat the oil in a large nonstick skillet over a medium-high temperature. Add onions and cook for about 3-4 minutes, or until translucent. Stir in garlic, thyme and about 2 tablespoons of water. Cook for 2 minutes and add squash, zucchini, and chickpeas. Cook for another 10 minutes, or until squash and zucchini are fork-tender. Stir occasionally.

Reduce the heat to low and add bulgur. Stir well to combine and cover with a lid. Cook for 10 more minutes. Remove from the heat and sprinkle with basil, salt, and pepper, to taste. Serve warm.

Nutrition information per serving: Kcal: 386, Protein: 17.3g, Carbs: 70.2g, Fats: 6.1g

JUICES

1.   Cabbage Orange Juice

Ingredients:

1 cup of purple cabbage, torn

1 large orange, peeled

1 cup of papaya, chopped

1 cup of goji berries

1 tsp of ginger, ground

1 tsp of honey

Preparation:

Wash the cabbage thoroughly and torn with hands. Set aside.

Peel the orange and divide into wedges. Set aside.

Peel the papaya and cut lengthwise in half. Scoop out the black seeds and flesh using a spoon. Cut into small chunks and set aside.

Place the goji berries in a bowl and add 1 cup of water. Soak for 30 minutes before juicing.

Combine cabbage, orange, papaya, and goji berries in a juicer and process until juiced.

Transfer to serving glasses and stir in the ginger and honey.

Add some ice cubes and serve immediately.

Nutritional information per serving: Kcal: 172, Protein: 4.3g, Carbs: 54.2g, Fats: 0.7g

2.   Basil Celery Juice

Ingredients:

1 cup of fresh basil

1 cup of fresh celery, chopped

2 large tomatoes, chopped

½ tsp of salt

½ tsp of dried oregano, ground

Preparation:

Combine basil and celery in a colander and wash under cold running water. Torn with hands and set aside.

Wash the tomatoes and place them in a bowl. Cut into quarters and reserve the juice while cutting. Set aside.

Now, combine basil, celery, and tomatoes in a juicer and process until juiced.

Transfer to serving glasses and stir in the reserved tomato juice, salt. Sprinkle with some oregano for some extra taste.

Refrigerate for 5 minutes before serving.

Nutrition information per serving: Kcal: 64, Protein: 4.6g, Carbs: 17.8g, Fats: 1.1g

3.   Beet Apple Juice

Ingredients:

1 cup of beets, trimmed

1 large red apple, cored

1 cup of fresh strawberries

1 large lime, peeled

1 ginger root knob, 1-inch

1 tbsp of liquid honey

2 oz of water

Preparation:

Wash the beets and trim off the green parts. Cut into small pieces and fill the measuring cup. Reserve the beet greens for some other juice. Set aside.

Wash the apple and remove the core. Cut into bite-sized pieces. Set aside.

Place the strawberries in a colander and wash under cold running water. Drain and cut in half. Set aside.

Peel the lime and cut lengthwise in half. Set aside.

Peel the ginger root knob and set aside.

Now, combine beets, apple, strawberries, and ginger in a juicer and process until juiced. Transfer to serving glasses and stir in honey and water.

Add some ice and serve immediately.

Nutrition information per serving: Kcal: 277, Protein: 4.2g, Carbs: 82.4g, Fats: 1.3g

4.　　Lime Melon Juice

Ingredients:

1 large lime, peeled

2 large honeydew melon wedges

1 cup of fresh mint, torn

1 large yellow apple, cored

2 oz of coconut water

Preparation:

Peel the lime and cut lengthwise in half. Set aside.

Cut the honeydew melon lengthwise in half. Scoop out the seeds using a spoon. Cut two large wedges and peel them. Cut into small chunks and place in a bowl. Wrap the rest of the melon in a plastic foil and refrigerate.

Wash the mint thoroughly under cold running water. Drain and torn with hands. Set aside.

Wash the apple and remove the core. Cut into bite-sized pieces and set aside.

Now, combine lime, honeydew melon, mint, and apple in a juicer. Transfer to serving glasses and stir in the coconut water.

Add some ice and serve immediately.

Nutrition information per serving: Kcal: 228, Protein: 3.4g, Carbs: 65.7g, Fats: 1g

5.   Cabbage Beet Juice

Ingredients:

1 cup of purple cabbage, chopped

1 large beet, trimmed

1 cup of pineapple chunks

1 large carrot, sliced

1 cup of fresh spinach, torn

1 tbsp of liquid honey

Preparation:

Cut the top of a pineapple and peel it using a sharp knife. Cut into small chunks and fill the measuring cup. Reserve the rest of the pineapple in a refrigerator.

Wash the purple cabbage and spinach thoroughly torn with hands. Set aside.

Wash the beet and trim off the green parts. Cut into small pieces and set aside.

Wash the carrot and cut into thick slices. Set aside.

Now, combine cabbage, beet, pineapple, carrot, and spinach in a juicer and process until juiced.

Transfer to serving glasses and stir in the liquid honey. Add few ice cubes and serve immediately.

Enjoy!

Nutrition information per serving: Kcal: 205, Protein: 5g, Carbs: 62.1g, Fats: 0.7g

6.   Swiss Chard Cucumber Juice

Ingredients:

1 cup of fresh parsley, torn

2 cups of Swiss chard, torn

1 large cucumber, sliced

1 small yellow apple, cored

1 small orange, peeled

Preparation:

Combine Swiss chard and parsley in a colander and wash thoroughly under cold running water. Drain and torn with hands. Set aside.

Wash the cucumber and cut into thick slices. Set aside.

Wash the apple and remove the core. Cut into bite-sized pieces and set aside.

Peel the orange and divide into wedges. Set aside.

Now, combine Swiss chard, cucumber, parsley, apple, and orange in a juicer and process until juiced. Transfer to serving glasses and add some ice before serving.

Enjoy!

Nutrition information per serving: Kcal: 161, Protein: 6.3g, Carbs: 46.3g, Fats: 1.2g

7.   Green Orange Juice

Ingredients:

1 cup of collard greens, chopped

1 cup of Swiss chard, chopped

1 large orange, peeled

1 cup of red leaf lettuce, chopped

1 cup of Romaine lettuce, chopped

1 large cucumber

1 large lemon, peeled

2 oz of water

Preparation:

Combine collard greens, Swiss chard, red leaf lettuce, and Romaine lettuce in a colander. Wash under cold running water and drain. Torn with hands and set aside.

Peel the orange and divide into wedges. Set aside.

Wash the cucumber and cut into thick slices. Set aside.

Peel the lemon and cut lengthwise in half. Set aside.

Now, combine collard greens, Swiss chard, orange, red leaf

lettuce, Romaine lettuce, cucumber, and lemon in a juicer and process until juiced.

Transfer to serving glasses and stir in the water.

Add some ice and serve immediately.

Nutrition information per serving: Kcal: 136, Protein: 7g, Carbs: 43.4g, Fats: 1.2g

8.   Beet Radish Juice

Ingredients:

1 cup of beets, trimmed and chopped

1 large radish, chopped

1 large orange, peeled

1 cup of fresh kale, chopped

1 large cucumber

Preparation:

Wash the beets and trim off the green parts. Chop into bite-sized pieces and set aside.

Wash the radish and trim off the green parts. Cut into small pieces and set aside.

Peel the orange and divide into wedges. Set aside.

Wash the kale thoroughly under cold running water. Drain and torn with hands. Set aside.

Wash the cucumber and cut into thick slices. Set aside.

Now, combine beets, radish, orange, kale, and cucumber in a juicer and process until juiced.

Transfer to serving glasses and add some ice before serving.

Enjoy!

Nutrition information per serving: Kcal: 174, Protein: 8.8g, Carbs: 51.7g, Fats: 1.4g

9. Tomato Swiss Chard Juice

Ingredients:

1 large tomato, chopped

1 cup of Swiss chard, torn

1 cup of asparagus, trimmed

1 cup of Brussels sprouts, trimmed

1 large cucumbers, sliced

Preparation:

Wash the tomato and place in a bowl. Cut into quarters and reserve the juice while cutting. Set aside.

Wash the Swiss chard thoroughly under cold running water. Drain and set aside.

Wash the asparagus and trim off the woody ends. Cut into 1-inch pieces and set aside.

Wash the Brussels sprouts and trim off the outer layers. Cut in half and set aside.

Wash the cucumber and cut into thick slices. Set aside.

Now, combine tomato, Swiss chard, asparagus, Brussels sprouts, and cucumber in a juicer and process until juiced.

Transfer to serving glasses and add some ice before serving.

Nutrition information per serving: Kcal: 109, Protein: 10.1g, Carbs: 32.4g, Fats: 1.2g

10.   Avocado Cucumber Juice

Ingredients:

1 cup of avocado, chopped

1 large cucumber, sliced

1 large tomato, chopped

1 large lemon, peeled

1 cup of fresh basil, chopped

Preparation:

Peel the avocado and cut in half. Remove the pit and cut into chunks. Fill the measuring cup and reserve the rest for some other juice. Keep it in a refrigerator.

Wash the cucumber and cut into thick slices. Set aside.

Wash the tomato and place in a bowl. Cut into quarters and reserve the juice while cutting. Set aside.

Peel the lemon and cut lengthwise in half. Set aside.

Wash the basil thoroughly and roughly chop it. Set aside.

Now, combine avocado, cucumber, tomato, lemon and basil in a juicer and process until juiced.

Transfer to serving glasses and add some ice before serving.

Enjoy!

Nutrition information per serving: Kcal: 240, Protein: 3.1g, Carbs: 75.1g, Fats: 0.9g

11.   Coconut Squash Juice

Ingredients:

½ cup of coconut water, unsweetened

1 cup of butternut squash, chunked

1 medium-sized banana, peeled

1 cup of raspberries, fresh

1 tsp of honey, raw

Preparation:

Peel the butternut squash and remove the seeds using a spoon. Cut into small cubes and reserve the rest of the squash for some other recipe. Wrap in a plastic foil and refrigerate.

Peel the banana and cut into chunks. Set aside.

Wash the raspberries under cold running water. Drain and set aside.

Now, combine butternut squash, banana, and raspberries in a juicer. Transfer to serving glasses and stir in the coconut water and honey.

Add some ice and serve immediately.

Enjoy!

Nutritional information per serving: Kcal: 197, Protein: 4.7g, Carbs: 68g, Fats: 1.3g

12.   Cranberry Coconut Juice

Ingredients:

1 cup of cranberries

3 oz of coconut water

1 cup of blackberries

1 cup of blueberries

1 cup of strawberries, chopped

1 cup of raspberries

Preparation:

Combine cranberries, blackberries, blueberries, strawberries, and raspberries in a large colander. Rinse well under cold running water. Drain and separate the strawberries.

Cut the strawberries into bite-sized pieces and set aside.

Now, combine all in a juicer and process until juiced. Transfer to serving glasses and add some ice before serving. Optionally, add some honey for some extra taste.

Enjoy!

Nutrition information per serving: Kcal: 210, Protein: 5.9g, Carbs: 75.3g, Fats: 2.5g

13.   Lettuce Orange Juice

Ingredients:

3 cups of red leaf lettuce, torn

1 large orange, peeled

1 cup of avocado, sliced

½ cup of pure coconut water, unsweetened

1 tsp of liquid honey

Preparation:

Wash the lettuce thoroughly under cold running water. Torn with hands and set aside.

Peel the orange and divide into wedges. Set aside.

Peel the avocado and cut in half. Remove the pit and chop into chunks. Fill the measuring cup and reserve the rest for some other juice. Set aside.

Now, combine lettuce, orange, and avocado in a juicer and process until juiced.

Transfer to serving glasses and refrigerate for 5 minutes before serving.

Enjoy!

Nutrition information per serving: Kcal: 240, Protein: 4.9g, Carbs: 25.6g, Fats: 21.7g

14.   Brussels Sprout Carrot Juice

Ingredients:

1 cup of Brussels sprouts, chopped

1 cup of carrots, sliced

1 cup of broccoli, chopped

1 cup of turnip greens, chopped

4 large oranges, peeled

1 tbsp of honey

¼ cup of pure coconut water

Preparation:

Wash the Brussels sprouts and trim off the outer layers. Cut in half and set aside.

Wash the carrots and cut into thin slices. Set aside.

Wash the broccoli and cut into small pieces. Set aside.

Wash the turnip greens thoroughly and torn with hands. Set aside.

Peel the oranges and divide into wedges. Set aside.

Now, combine broccoli, Brussels sprouts, carrots, turnip

greens, and oranges in a juicer and process until juiced. Transfer to serving glasses and stir in the honey and coconut water.

Add some ice cubes before serving or refrigerate for 5 minutes.

Enjoy!

Nutrition information per serving: Kcal: 367, Protein: 14.47g, Carbs: 116g, Fats: 1.9g

15.   Kiwi Spinach Juice

Ingredients:

1 large kiwi, peeled

1 cup of fresh spinach, chopped

5 apricots, sliced

1 large peach, sliced

1 tbsp of fresh mint, chopped

¼ cup of water

Preparation:

Peel the kiwi and cut lengthwise in half. Set aside.

Wash the spinach and mint under cold running water. Drain and roughly chop it. Set aside.

Wash the apricots and cut in half. Remove the pits and cut into chunks. Set aside.

Wash the peach and cut in half. Remove the pit and cut into small pieces. Set aside.

Now, combine kiwi, spinach, apricots, peach, and mint in a juicer and process until juiced.

Transfer to serving glasses and refrigerate before serving.

Nutrition information per serving: Kcal: 211, Protein: 2.8g, Carbs: 58.8g, Fats: 2.8g

16.   Lime Broccoli Juice

Ingredients:

2 whole limes, peeled

2 cups of raw broccoli, chopped

1 cup of fresh raspberries

½ cup of coconut water, unsweetened

2 large cucumbers, peeled and sliced

1 tbsp of honey

Preparation:

Peel the limes and cut lengthwise in half. Set aside.

Wash the broccoli and cut into small pieces. Set aside.

Wash the raspberries under cold running water. Drain and set aside.

Wash the cucumbers and cut into thick slices. Set aside.

Combine limes, broccoli, raspberries, and cucumber in a juicer and process until juiced. Transfer to serving glasses and stir in the coconut water and honey.

Add some ice and serve.

Nutritional information per serving: Kcal: 192, Protein: 10.9g, Carbs: 56g, Fats: 2.2g

17.   Radish Swiss Chard Juice

Ingredients:

1 large radish, chopped

1 cup of Swiss chard, torn

1 large honeydew melon wedge

1 cup of asparagus

1 cup of avocado, chopped

¼ cup of pure coconut water, unsweetened

Preparation:

Wash the radish and trim off the green parts. Cut into small pieces and set aside.

Wash the chard thoroughly and torn with hands. Set aside.

Cut the honeydew melon lengthwise in half. Scoop out the seeds using a spoon. Cut the large wedges and peel them. Cut into small chunks and place in a bowl. Wrap the rest of the melon in a plastic foil and refrigerate.

Wash the asparagus and trim off the woody ends. Chop into small pieces and set aside.

Peel the avocado and cut in half. Remove the pit and cut

into chunks. Set aside.

Now, combine radish, chard, melon, asparagus, and avocado in a juicer and process until juiced.

Transfer to serving glasses and refrigerate 10 minutes before serving.

Nutritional information per serving: Kcal: 275, Protein: 8g, Carbs: 35.2g, Fats: 21,9g

18.   Coconut Guava Juice

Ingredients:

1 large guava, chopped

¼ cup of pure coconut water, unsweetened

1 tbsp of pure coconut sugar

1 small ginger root slice, peeled and chopped

2 cups of Swiss chard, torn

2 cups of fresh kale, torn

A bunch of spinach, torn

Preparation:

Wash the guava and cut into chunks. Set aside.

Peel the ginger slice and set aside.

Combine Swiss chard, kale, and spinach in a colander and wash thoroughly under cold running water. Drain and torn with hands. Set aside.

Now, combine guava, ginger, Swiss chard, kale, and spinach in a juicer and process until juiced.

Transfer to serving glasses and stir in the coconut water

and pure coconut sugar.

Add some ice and serve immediately.

Nutrition information per serving: Kcal: 267, Protein: 22.3g, Carbs: 45g, Fats: 3.8g

19. Nutmeg Apple Juice

Ingredients:

1 small apple, peeled and seeds removed

1 cup of pineapple, chunked

1 tsp of fresh mint leaves, finely chopped

¼ tsp of nutmeg, ground

Preparation:

Wash the apple and remove the core. Cut into bite-sized pieces and set aside.

Cut the top of a pineapple and peel it using a sharp knife. Cut into small chunks. Reserve the rest of the pineapple in a refrigerator.

Combine apple and pineapple and process in a juicer. Transfer to a serving glasses and stir in the nutmeg. Add more water to increase the juice amount.

Garnish with mint leaves and refrigerate before serving.

Nutritional information per serving: Kcal: 141, Protein: 1.5g, Carbs: 41.2g, Fats: 0.4g

20. Blueberry Carrot Juice

Ingredients:

1 cup of fresh blueberries

2 large carrots, sliced

1 small apple, cored and chopped

1 head romaine lettuce, torn

Preparation:

Wash the blueberries under cold running water. Set aside aside.

Wash the carrots and cut into thick slices. Set aside.

Wash the apple and remove the core. Cut into bite-sized pieces and set aside.

Wash the lettuce thoroughly and torn with hands. Set aside.

Now, process blueberries, carrots, apple, and lettuce in a juicer. Transfer to serving glasses and add few ice cubes.

Serve immediately.

Nutritional information per serving: Kcal: 228, Protein: 6.14g, Carbs: 66.8g, Fats: 1.95g

21. Grape Orange Juice

Ingredients:

½ cup of fresh grapes

3 large oranges, peeled

1 medium-sized pear, roughly chopped

1 cup of spinach, torn

1 small ginger root slice, peeled

Preparation:

Wash the grapes in a colander under cold running water and set aside.

Peel the oranges and divide into wedges. Set aside.

Wash the pear and remove the core. Cut into small pieces and set aside.

Wash the spinach thoroughly and torn with hands. Set aside.

Peel the ginger slice and set aside.

Combine grapes, oranges, pear, spinach, and ginger in a juicer and process until juiced.

Transfer to serving glasses and refrigerate for 10 minutes before serving.

Enjoy!

Nutritional information per serving: Kcal: 347, Protein: 6.52g, Carbs: 108.8g, Fats: 1.27g

22.   Sweet Banana Orange Juice

Ingredients:

1 large banana, peeled

1 large orange, peeled

1 cup of parsnips, sliced

1 cup of cauliflower, chopped

A handful of fresh mint, chopped

1 tsp of honey, raw

Preparation:

Peel the banana and cut into chunks. Set aside.

Peel the orange and divide into wedges. Set aside.

Wash the parsnips and cut into thick slices. Set aside.

Trim off the outer leaves of cauliflower. Wash it and cut into small pieces. Reserve the rest in the refrigerator.

Now, combine banana, orange, parsnips, and cauliflower in a juicer and process until juiced. Transfer to serving glasses and stir in the honey. Sprinkle with mint and refrigerate for 5 minutes before serving.

Enjoy!

Nutritional information per serving: Kcal: 336, Protein: 8.5g, Carbs: 103g, Fats: 1.5g

23.   Coconut Lemon Juice

Ingredients:

½ cup of coconut water, unsweetened

2 large lemons, peeled

1 cup of broccoli, chopped

A bunch of fresh spinach

1 medium-sized orange

1 tbsp of honey, raw

A few mint leaves

Preparation:

Peel the lemons and cut lengthwise in half. Set aside.

Wash the broccoli and trim off the outer leaves. Set aside.

Wash the spinach thoroughly and torn with hands. Set aside.

Peel the orange and divide into wedges. Set aside.

Now, combine broccoli, spinach, lemons, and orange in a juicer and process until juiced. Transfer to serving glasses and stir in the honey and garnish with mint leaves.

Add some ice and serve.

Nutritional information per serving: Kcal: 171, Protein: 14.8g, Carbs: 54.5g, Fats: 2.17g

24.   Kale Cranberries Juice

Ingredients:

1 cup of kale, torn

1 cup of cranberries

3 large kiwis, peeled

1 tsp of pure coconut sugar

Preparation:

Wash the kale thoroughly and torn with hands. Set aside.

Wash the cranberries under cold running water. Drain and set aside.

Peel the kiwis and cut lengthwise in half. Set aside.

Now, combine kiwis, kale, and cranberries in a juicer. Transfer to serving glasses and stir in the coconut water.

Add some ice and serve!

Nutritional information per serving: Kcal: 153, Protein: 5.6g, Carbs: 48.4g, Fats: 1.8g

25.   Baby Spinach Ginger Juice

Ingredients:

¼ cup of baby spinach

½ tsp of ginger, ground

1 cup of blackberries

1 cup of blueberries

1 cup of raspberries

1 cup of strawberries, chopped

Preparation:

Wash the spinach thoroughly and torn with hands. Set aside.

Combine all berries in a colander and wash under cold running water. Set aside.

Now, mix all berries and spinach in a juicer and process until juiced. Transfer to serving glasses and stir in the ginger.

Add few ice cubes and serve immediately.

Enjoy!

Nutritional information per serving: Kcal: 158, Protein: 5.9g, Carbs: 56.4g, Fats: 2.3g

26. Grapefruit Honey Juice

Ingredients:

1 large grapefruit, peeled

1 tsp of honey, raw

2 large Granny Smith apples, cored and chopped

½ tsp of ginger, freshly ground

Preparation:

Wash the grapefruit and chop into small pieces. Set aside.

Wash the apples and remove the core. Chop into bite-sized pieces and set aside.

Combine grapefruit and apples and process in a juicer. Transfer to serving glasses and stir in the honey and ginger.

Refrigerate or add some ice and serve.

Enjoy!

Nutritional information per serving: Kcal: 299, Protein: 3.7g, Carbs: 88g, Fats: 1.1g

27.   Spinach Banana Juice

Ingredients:

2 cups of spinach, chopped

1 medium-sized banana, sliced

2 cups of fresh strawberries, chopped

14 oz melon, roughly chopped

½ tsp of cinnamon

1 tsp of honey, raw

Preparation:

Wash the spinach thoroughly and torn with hands. Set aside.

Peel the banana and cut into small chunks. Set aside.

Wash the strawberries under cold running water and chop into small pieces. Set aside.

Cut the melon in half. Cut two large wedges and peel. Cut into small chunks and remove the seeds. Set aside.

Now, combine spinach, banana, strawberries, and melon in a juicer and process until juiced. Transfer to serving glasses and stir in the honey and cinnamon.

Refrigerate for 5 minutes before serving minutes.

Nutritional information per serving: Kcal: 349, Protein: 7.6g, Carbs: 104.9g, Fats: 3.2g

28.   Pineapple Mango Juice

Ingredients:

1 cup of pineapple chopped

1 cup of mango, chopped

½ cup of coconut water

1 cup of guava, chopped

1 tbsp of fresh mint leaves

Preparation:

Cut the top of a pineapple and peel it using a sharp knife. Cut into small pieces. Reserve the rest of the pineapple in a refrigerator.

Peel the mango and cut into small pieces. Set aside.

Wash the guava and cut into pieces. If you are using large fruit, reserve the rest for some other recipe in a refrigerator.

Now, combine pineapple, mango, and guava in a juicer.

Transfer to serving glasses and stir in the coconut water.

Garnish with some mint leaves and add some ice before serving.

Enjoy!

Nutritional information per serving: Kcal: 187, Protein: 3.6g, Carbs: 54.2g, Fats: 1.3g

29.   Blueberry Coconut Juice

Ingredients:

1 cup of blueberries

½ cup of coconut water, unsweetened

2 cups of strawberries, chopped

½ large red orange

1 tsp of pure coconut sugar

Preparation:

Combine blueberries and strawberries in a colander and wash under cold running water. Set aside.

Peel the orange and divide into wedges. Use about half of the wedges and reserve the rest for some other juice.

Combine blueberries, strawberries, and orange in a juicer. Transfer to serving glasses and stir in the coconut water and coconut sugar.

Add some ice or refrigerate before serving.

Nutritional information per serving: Kcal: 246, Protein: 4.7g, Carbs: 74.2g, Fats: 1.7g

30. Raspberry Blueberry Juice

Ingredients:

2 cups of raspberries

1 cup of blueberries

½ cup of coconut water, unsweetened

½ tsp of pure vanilla extract, sugar-free

¼ tsp of cinnamon, ground

Preparation:

Wash the raspberries and blueberries under cold running water. Drain well. Transfer all to a juicer and process until juiced.

Transfer to serving glasses and stir in the coconut water, vanilla extract, and cinnamon.

Add few ice cubes and serve immediately.

Enjoy!

Nutritional information per serving: Kcal: 136, Protein: 4.4g, Carbs: 51.7g, Fats: 2.4g

31.   Beet Tomato Juice

Ingredients:

1 cup of beets

3 large tomatoes, peeled

2 large apples, cored and peeled

1 cup of goji berries

1 cup of fresh cherries, pitted

Preparation:

Wash the beets and trim off the green parts. Cut into small pieces and set aside.

Place the tomatoes in a bowl and chop into quarters. Reserve the juice while cutting.

Wash the cherries and remove the pits. Set aside.

Wash the apples and remove the core. Cut into bite-sized pieces and set aside.

Place the goji berries in a medium bowl and add 1 cup of water. Soak for 30 minutes before juicing.

Now, combine apples, goji berries, beets, cherries, and tomatoes in a juicer.

Transfer to serving glasses and stir in the reserved tomato juice.

Refrigerate for 10 minutes before serving.

Nutritional information per serving: Kcal: 328, Protein: 9.3g, Carbs: 95g, Fats: 2.14g

32.   Orange Goji Juice

Ingredients:

1 large orange, peeled

1 cup of goji berries

10 oz broccoli, pre-cooked

1 large cucumber, peeled

1 tbsp of honey, raw

Preparation:

Peel the orange and divide into wedges. Set aside.

Place the goji berries in a medium bowl. Add 1 cup of water and soak for 30 minutes.

Wash the broccoli and chop into small pieces. Set aside.

Wash the cucumber and cut into thick slices. Set aside.

Now, process orange, goji berries, broccoli, and cucumber in a juicer. Transfer to serving glasses and stir in the honey.

Add some ice and serve!

Nutritional information per serving: Kcal: 193, Protein: 9.4g, Carbs: 66g, Fats: 1.7g

33.   Banana Honey Juice

Ingredients:

1 large banana, peeled

1 tsp of honey

1 cup of blueberries

1 cup of blackberries

½ tsp of cinnamon

Preparation:

Peel the banana and chop into chunks. Set aside.

Combine blueberries and blackberries in a colander and wash under cold running water. Drain and set aside. Now, combine banana, blueberries, and blackberries in a juicer and process until juiced. Transfer to serving glasses and stir in the honey and cinnamon.

Add some ice and serve immediately.

Nutritional information per serving: Kcal: 229, Protein: 4.5g, Carbs: 76.3g, Fats: 1.6g

34.   Tangerine Coffee Juice

Ingredients:

4 whole tangerines, peeled and wedged

½ cup of chilled coffee

1 tsp of pure vanilla extract

1 tsp of pure coconut sugar

Preparation:

Peel the tangerines and divide into wedges. Set aside. Run through a juicer and transfer to serving glasses.

Stir in the chilled coffee, coconut sugar, and vanilla extract.

Add some ice cubes and serve immediately.

Nutritional information per serving: Kcal: 282, Protein: 6.9g, Carbs: 94g, Fats: 2g

35. Banana Chokeberry Juice

Ingredients:

1 large banana, peeled

2 cups of chokeberries

2 cups of spinach, torn

2 cups of beet greens, torn

Preparation:

Peel the banana and cut into chunks. Set aside.

Wash the chokeberries under cold running water using a colander. Drain and set aside.

Combine spinach and beet greens in a colander and wash thoroughly. Torn with hands and set aside. Now, combine banana, berries, spinach, and beet greens in a juicer. Transfer to serving glasses and add some ice cubes before serving.

Enjoy!

Nutritional information per serving: Kcal: 183, Protein: 7.8g, Carbs: 63.1g, Fats: 1.2g

36.   Pumpkin Cinnamon Juice

Ingredients:

10 oz of pumpkin, chopped

½ tsp of cinnamon, freshly ground

1 cup of sweet potato, chunked

¼ cup of water

Preparation:

Peel the pumpkin and cut in half. Scoop out the seeds and cut into small chunks. Set aside.

Peel the sweet potato and cut into bite-sized pieces. Set aside.

Now, combine pumpkin and sweet potato in a juicer and process until juiced.

Transfer to serving glasses and stir in the water and cinnamon.

Add some ice before serving and enjoy!

Nutritional information per serving: Kcal: 256, Protein: 5.3g, Carbs: 27.8g, Fats: 22.3g

37.   Carrot Apple Juice

Ingredients:

3 large carrots, sliced

2 Granny Smith's apples, cored and chopped

½ tsp of cinnamon, freshly ground

¼ tsp of ginger, ground

1 tbsp of honey, raw

Preparation:

Wash the carrots and chop into thick slices. Set aside.

Wash the apples and remove the core. Cut into bite-sized pieces and set aside.

Combine carrots and apples in a juicer and process until juiced. Transfer to serving glasses and stir in the honey, cinnamon, and ginger.

Add few ice cubes and serve immediately.

Nutritional information per serving: Kcal: 324, Protein: 3.4g, Carbs: 93g, Fats: 1.5g

38.   Grape Vanilla Juice

Ingredients:

1 cup of grapes

1 tsp of pure vanilla extract, sugar-free

2 large bananas, sliced

½ cup of coconut milk, sugar-free

Preparation:

Wash the grapes under cold running water. Drain and set aside.

Peel the bananas and chop into small chunks. Set aside.

Combine bananas and grapes in a juicer and process until juiced. Transfer to serving glasses and stir in the coconut milk and vanilla extract.

Add some ice and serve!

Nutritional information per serving: Kcal: 293, Protein: 7.5g, Carbs: 77.9g, Fats: 4g

39.   Cucumber Grapefruit Juice

Ingredients:

3 large cucumbers, peeled

1 grapefruit, peeled

1 tsp of peppermint extract

1 oz of coconut water

1 tbsp of coconut sugar

Preparation:

Wash the cucumbers and cut into thick slices. Set aside.

Peel the grapefruit and cut into bite-sized pieces. set aside. Now, combine cucumber and grapefruit in a juicer and process until juiced. Transfer to serving glasses and stir in the coconut water, coconut sugar and peppermint extract. Add some ice cubes and serve immediately.

Nutritional information per serving: Kcal: 204, Protein: 7.7g, Carbs: 59g, Fats: 1.3g

40. Flaxseed Banana Juice

Ingredients:

1 tsp of flaxseed oil

1 large banana

1 cup of goji berries

A bunch of celery leaves

1 tbsp of honey, raw

Preparation:

Peel the banana and cut into small chunks. Set aside.

Place the goji berries in a medium bowl and add 1 cup of water. Soak for 30 minutes. Wash the celery and torn with hands. Set aside. Now, combine banana, goji berries, and celery in a juicer and process until juiced. Transfer to serving glasses and stir in the flaxseed oil and honey. Add few ice cubes before serving.

Nutritional information per serving: Kcal: 177, Protein: 6.5g, Carbs: 44.6g, Fats: 2.6g

41.   Raspberry Cherry Juice

Ingredients:

1 cup of fresh raspberries

½ tsp of pure cherry extract, sugar-free

1 large cucumber, sliced

A couple of mint leaves

Preparation:

Wash the raspberries under cold running water. Drain and set aside.

Wash the cucumber and cut into thin slices. Set aside.

Combine raspberries and cucumber in a juicer and process until juiced. Transfer to serving glasses and stir in the cherry extract.

Garnish with fresh mint leaves and refrigerate for 10 minutes before serving.

Nutritional information per serving: Kcal: 152, Protein: 9.4g, Carbs: 50g, Fats: 2.6g

42.   Blackberry Cucumber Juice

Ingredients:

1 cup of fresh blackberries

1 large cucumber, sliced

1 cup of pomegranate seeds

1 cup of fresh parsley

Preparation:

Wash the blackberries under cold running water. Drain and set aside.

Wash the cucumber and cut into thick slices. Set aside.

Cut the top of the pomegranate fruit using a sharp knife. Slice down to each of the white membranes inside of the fruit. Pop the seeds into a medium bowl.

Wash the parsley thoroughly and roughly chop with hands. Set aside.

Now, combine blackberries, cucumber, pomegranate seeds, and parsley.

Transfer to serving glasses and add some ice cubes before serving.

Nutritional information per serving: Kcal: 143, Protein: 7.9g, Carbs: 44.8g, Fats: 2.5g

43.   Strawberry Ginger Juice

Ingredients:

1 cup of strawberries, fresh

½ tsp of ginger, ground

1 cup of fresh kale, torn

1 whole lemon, peeled

Preparation:

Wash the strawberries under cold running water. Drain and set aside.

Wash the kale thoroughly and torn with hands. Set aside. Peel the lemon and cut lengthwise in half. Set aside. Combine strawberries, kale, and lemon in a juicer and process until juiced.

Transfer to serving glasses add some ice cubes before serving.

Enjoy!

Nutritional information per serving: Kcal: 120, Protein: 5.9g, Carbs: 38.6g, Fats: 1.8g

44.   Parsnip Celery Juice

Ingredients:

1 cup of parsnips, chopped

1 celery stalk, chopped

1 whole guava, chopped

2 large grapefruits, peeled

Preparation:

Wash the parsnips and cut into small slices. Set aside.

Wash the celery and cut into small pieces. Set aside.

Wash the guava and cut into chunks. If you are using large fruit, reserve the rest for some other recipe in a refrigerator. Peel the grapefruits and chop into bite-sized pieces. Now, combine parsnips, celery, guava, and grapefruits in a juicer and process until juiced. Transfer to serving glasses and add some ice before serving.

Nutritional information per serving: Kcal: 279, Protein: 7.2g, Carbs: 86g, Fats: 1.7g

45. Carrot Parsnip Juice

Ingredients:

2 large green apples, peeled and cored

3 large carrots, sliced

1 cup of parsnips, sliced

1 basil leaf, crushed

¼ cup of water

Preparation:

Wash the carrots and parsnips and cut into thick slices. Set aside.

Wash the apples and remove the core. Cut into bite-sized pieces and set aside. Now, combine carrots, parsnips, and apples in a juicer and process until juiced. Transfer to serving glasses and stir in the water. Garnish with basil leaves and refrigerate before serving.

Nutritional information per serving: Kcal: 332, Protein: 5.4g, Carbs: 100g, Fats: 1.6g

46.   Artichoke Lemon Juice

Ingredients:

7 oz of artichokes, chopped

1 medium-sized lemon, peeled

1 whole avocado, chopped

1 cup of red cabbage, torn

1 cup of green cabbage, torn

Preparation:

Trim off the outer leaves of the artichoke using a sharp knife. Cut into small pieces and set aside.

Peel the lemon and cut lengthwise in half. Set aside.

Peel the avocado and cut in half. Remove the pit and cut into chunks. Set aside.

Combine red and green cabbage in a colander and wash under cold running water. Drain and torn with hands. Set aside.

Now, combine artichoke, lemon, avocado, and cabbages in a juicer and process until juiced.

Transfer to serving glasses and add some ice before

serving.

Enjoy!

Nutritional information per serving: Kcal: 353, Protein: 12.3g, Carbs: 51g, Fats: 30g

ADDITIONAL TITLES FROM THIS AUTHOR

70 Effective Meal Recipes to Prevent and Solve Being Overweight: Burn Fat Fast by Using Proper Dieting and Smart Nutrition

By

Joe Correa CSN

48 Acne Solving Meal Recipes: The Fast and Natural Path to Fixing Your Acne Problems in Less Than 10 Days!

By

Joe Correa CSN

41 Alzheimer's Preventing Meal Recipes: Reduce or Eliminate Your Alzheimer's Condition in 30 Days or Less!

By

Joe Correa CSN

70 Effective Breast Cancer Meal Recipes: Prevent and Fight Breast Cancer with Smart Nutrition and Powerful Foods

By

Joe Correa CSN

www.ingramcontent.com/pod-product-compliance
Lightning Source LLC
Chambersburg PA
CBHW030250030426
42336CB00009B/330